MEN'S SKIN HEALTH

SKIN SOLUTIONS TO OVERCOME DRY SKIN AND
KEEP YOUR LARGEST ORGAN HEALTHY FROM
HEAD TO TOE AND EVERY INCH IN BETWEEN

GREGORY LANDSMAN

CONTENTS

Published in the United States by Hill of Content Publishing

Published in the United Kingdom by Hill of Content Publishing

Published in Australia by Hill of Content Publishing

Published in India by Hill of Content Publishing

hillofcontentpublishing.com

PO Box 24 East Melbourne 8002 Victoria Australia

Distributed by Etoile International Group. Hong Kong.

Design and images: Angela Brille and Rose Hart

National Library of Australia Cataloguing-in-Publication data:

Landsman, Gregory
Men's Skin Health

Includes index: ISBN: 978-0-6483443-7-7

Every day we get up to fight the good fight
We rise to a challenge and take risks when we need to
We work hard and play hard
We learn from our mistakes and live each day with no regrets
We love and we laugh
We know when to hold on and when to move on
We do what we need to get the job done
We won't give up if we can still stand up
We know what matters in life and we treasure it
We think in terms of possibilities and push past our limits
We make the most of who we are and strive to be our best

Gregory Landsman

MEN'S SKIN IS UNDER ATTACK

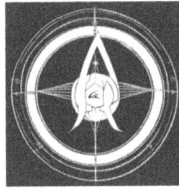

In my work with people across the globe - in wellness centres, my treatment room in Geneva and within the fashion and beauty industry, it has become apparent that chronically dry skin is becoming more and more of an issue for men.

Men's skin is under attack from head to toe and every inch in between, and while we are doing all we can to address the symptoms, often we are unaware of the cause.

Recently, the GL Skinfit Institute undertook research with more than 5000 men in the USA and Australia about their experiences with skin dryness.

The outcome of this research showed that men are suffering from dry skin for longer periods and more often; and that the age group experiencing dry skin regularly or ongoing is widening to encompass the 25-40 age group in larger numbers.

It also indicated that while dry skin often showed on their faces, that one of the primary areas where dry skin had become a genuine issue, and not just a mild irritation, was on their penile skin.

THE QUESTION IS WHY?

This book provides insights and solutions to the day-to-day impact of lifestyle choices and environment that dry, stress and prematurely age the skin.

But more importantly, we look at the rarely discussed underlying causes of dry skin in many men - stress, low T-levels, and diet.

THE 'SKIN – STRESS – T-LEVEL' CONNECTION?

In many cases the real culprit is what I call the 'Skin-Stress-Testosterone' connection. Our largest organ, our skin, makes up around sixteen percent of our total weight and is a ruthless indicator of our stress levels, our lifestyle choices, our T-levels and our overall health.

STRESS ATTACKS AND WEAKENS SKIN

Stress is a toothy beast that can eat us from the inside out. Feeling stressed is something that we have all learned to live with, but it can dry and age the skin, adding years to the look of our skin prematurely.

However, this doesn't just happen on our faces, it impacts our entire body, including our skin below the belt, which is some of the most sensitive on the body.

STRESS LOWERS TESTOSTERONE LEVELS

But this isn't the only significant downside of living with ongoing stress. What is not often discussed is how the stress hormone that impacts skin, also significantly lowers men's testosterone, which at normal levels supports us to maintain healthy skin.

STRESS AND LOW T-LEVELS BOTH DRY THE SKIN

However, low testosterone levels consistently result in skin dryness – not just on the face, but the entire body. This often impacts the most sensitive skin areas first – leaving the skin feeling tight, uncomfortable and irritated.

There is a strong link between the impact that stress has on healthy skin and maintaining vital testosterone levels. But the connection doesn't stop there.

POSITIVE LIFESTYLE BEHAVIOURS SUPPORT GOOD SKIN, LOW STRESS AND OPTIMAL T-LEVELS

The lifestyle behaviours that naturally support healthy skin – the foods we eat; quality of sleep; mindfulness practices; and approaches to exercise, water and toxins – also support lower stress levels and healthy testosterone levels.

So by looking after our skin naturally through positive lifestyle choices, we can support healthy testosterone levels and lower stress levels.

This is great news! We can keep our skin looking fresh and

healthy, feel calmer and keep our T-levels at optimal levels all at the same time!

Men's Skin Health has been put together to support men to keep the skin on every part of their body looking healthy at every age, while naturally supporting lower stress and optimal testosterone levels.

This book will help you discover the four pillars of skin health, providing genuine natural solutions from the inside out and the outside in to keep your skin stronger, firmer, healthier and more vital from head to toe.

Nature has provided us with everything we need to keep our skin looking healthy at every age. By feeding the skin the right mix of skin-building vitamins and minerals topically in skincare treatments, absorption of the key nutrients is as high as if taken orally, and more targeted and effective to the skin area where the treatment is being applied.

Discover how to:

1. Give your skin a break from the toxins of everyday life with natural skin boosting vitamin and mineral formulas.
2. Eat cortisol lowering foods to lower stress and increase testosterone.
3. Speed up lymphatic drainage and oxygenate the blood to enable more nutrients to be carried to the skin.
4. Use skin renewing foods to cook your way to brighter, healthier looking skin.

5. Create simple, easy, DIY science-based treatments to combat dry skin on every part of the body.
6. Control the stress hormone (cortisol).
7. Activate your youth enhancing hormone while you sleep.
8. Breathe and energise your skin, naturally reduce cortisol levels and increase testosterone levels.

With regular application, these practices can stop the daily attack on your skin and make a remarkable difference to your stress levels, your T-levels and support healthy, vital looking skin.

I have practised these techniques personally for many years and have shared them extensively in my books, my TV show, in wellness centres and with clients.

However, please keep in mind that this book is not an alternative for medical advice, so if you are suffering from a serious skin or medical condition, please seek advice from your doctor before using any of these natural treatments.

Gregory Landsman
CEO , GL Skinfit Institute

GL FOUR PILLARS OF SKIN HEALTH

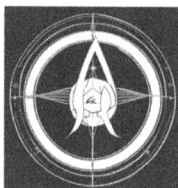

This book features techniques from each of my four pillars of skin health to provide you with a sustainable approach to maintaining skin health and vitality naturally at any age.

The key to maintaining skin health over a lifetime is to make small changes that can deliver big skin results when practised regularly.

Pillar 1: SKIN FOODS
The most powerful skin strengthening ingredients can be found in the foods we eat. By incorporating specific nutrient-rich foods into your diet, you can nourish your skin from the inside out, reduce stress and increase your T-levels.

Pillar 2: TOPICAL VITAMIN AND MINERAL FORMULAS
Renew your skin with topical vitamins and minerals from ingredients in your kitchen. You might be surprised to learn that you can renew your skin with powerful vitamins and minerals you can find right in your own kitchen. Many

common ingredients contain skin-boosting nutrients scientifically proven to enhance skin health and revive tired, dull skin.

Pillar 3: FACIAL MASSAGE AND EXERCISE
Rebuild skin health and vitality by strengthening the facial muscles and giving your face a good rub daily to increase lymphatic drainage, remove toxins and increase blood flow to the skin.

Pillar 4: BREATH WORK
While stress and day-to-day living can take a toll on our skin, one powerful tool that can have a positive impact on your skin's health and appearance is your breath. Changing the way you breathe can change not only your skin, but it will reduce the stress hormone by taking your body out of 'fight and flight' and into 'rest and digest'.
By taking time to change your breathing pattern you can help promote healthier, more vital looking skin from the inside out.

PART 1

MEN'S SKIN HEALTH

STRESS AND MEN'S SKIN

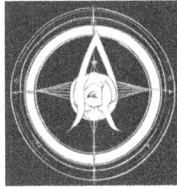

Since testosterone naturally declines with age and can be affected by many environmental factors, it's important to...

Eat healthy

Get seven to eight hours of sleep nightly

Limit alcohol to one drink per day

Quit smoking

Keep stress levels under control

All of these factors provide what is necessary for the body to produce optimal amounts of testosterone.

DR. CASTELLANOS, MD, PSYCHIATRIST CLINICAL
ASSISTANT PROFESSOR – HOFSTRA NORTH
SHORE-LIJ SCHOOL OF MEDICINE, NEW YORK

THE STRESS HORMONE THAT ATTACKS SKIN

Experts tell us that most of us are suffering from a state known as 'chronic stress' or stress that never goes away. As a result our faces, and every part of our bodies are suffering the impact of our higher stress levels.

When we are feeling stressed, the adrenal glands release the stress hormone known as cortisol. When this happens, sugar levels in the blood naturally increase, and the increased blood sugar promotes 'glycation' in our skin and damages our collagen. Damaged collagen equals an increase in skin dryness, wrinkles and premature aging.

Cortisol also decreases our skin's natural production of hyaluronic acid, which acts as a natural moisturiser for our skin. This allows even more hydration to be lost; and when skin is dehydrated, the enzymes in our skin that work to repair the damage don't work as well.

THE STRESS HORMONE IMPACTS TESTOSTERONE LEVELS

The release of cortisol into our bodies when we are under stress also inhibits the production of testosterone. A state of chronic stress means we are living with high levels of cortisol in our system, placing our healthy levels of testosterone under threat.

The body produces an enzyme to defend testosterone molecules from cortisol. However, when a man is suffering from ongoing stress, there is simply too much cortisol for this protective enzyme to manage, which results in testosterone being destroyed in the testicles, before it is released into the bloodstream.

For men this is not good news, as testosterone has been linked to many important health functions in the body, and it is certainly not good news for our skin.

Testosterone is one of the major keys for healthy skin, so when we talk about repairing men's dry skin, we have to discuss our T-levels and the role it plays in maintaining healthy, vital skin.

T-LEVELS IMPACT COLLAGEN PRODUCTION

Testosterone plays a key element in the production of collagen in the body. Collagen is an important protein in the skin that keeps it firm and elastic and supports its structure.

When testosterone levels drop, collagen production also declines. Which means our skin loses elasticity and firmness and fine lines and wrinkles begin to form.

T LEVELS AND DRY SKIN

Testosterone controls the sebum levels in our body, which act as a moisture barrier, to ensure thicker, healthier looking skin. Low testosterone levels can result in thinner, dryer skin and premature aging. This of course also applies to penile skin, which may in part account for the growing number of men suffering from dry penile skin conditions.

T-LEVELS NATURALLY DECREASE WITH AGE

Men's skin health and testosterone health are both severely impacted by stress, causing the skin to dry, weaken and age prematurely.

Beginning at age 30, testosterone levels drop around 1 percent a year and continue to decline at an even faster rate after the age of 40. While this is normal, it impacts our overall health, including our skin health.

Testosterone levels are also negatively impacted by a number of lifestyle elements including:

- High alcohol intake
- Smoking
- Low quality food
- Over or under eating
- Weight gain
- Lack of or excessive exercise
- Lack of sleep

It turns out these factors also impact men's skin health causing premature skin aging.

However, men's skin health and maintaining normal testosterone levels can be positively impacted naturally at any age through better lifestyle choices.

The good news is that you can support your testosterone levels and get great skin from head to toe and every inch in between at the same time!

SLEEP SUPPORTS HEALTHY TESTOSTERONE LEVELS

Getting enough sleep is critical for strong T-levels but it is also great for your skin health.

Something powerful happens when we fall asleep... we release a youth activating hormone called the human growth hormone that gets to work.

This hormone builds us up and helps create thicker skin, giving us a more youthful appearance overall, stronger bones and increased muscle mass.

It is a part of normal tissue repair, helping to regenerate what has been broken down by day-to-day activities.

Sleep is the simplest way to bolster your way to healthy skin and help build your testosterone levels.

**WE NEED TO DE-STRESS
OUR SKIN, BODIES AND OUR MINDS
SO WE AGE LESS!**

Your body is your only true possession and you take yourself wherever you go.

2

REDUCE STRESS AND INCREASE TESTOSTERONE LEVELS WITH MINDFULNESS TECHNIQUES

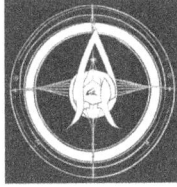

A simple breathing technique can instantly lower your stress levels.

DR. S. ADAM RAMIN, MD, UROLOGIST AND
MEDICAL DIRECTOR LOS ANGELES

THE FEEL GOOD FACTOR!

The first thing to understand is that a genuine solution to healthy skin that lasts the test of time is more than just waging war on frown lines and dry skin. A super healthy complexion is one that reflects the way we think, the way we eat and the way we live.

Looking and feeling our best is about using what nature has given us and then focusing on our quality of life, not just the quality of our skin.

BREATHING TO LOWER STRESS

Just taking a few minutes to breathe deeply every day can significantly lower stress and make you look and feel better. This is a simple technique that uses the abdominal muscles.

To start, simply breathe in through your nose, filling your stomach up with air. The sound of this deep breathing will remind you of gushing wind.

Hold your breath and then slowly exhale through your nose. As you exhale tighten the muscles of your stomach to push all air out of the lungs.

Focusing on your breath while breathing deeply releases endorphins throughout your body that make you feel good; provides the body with more energy through the increase in blood flow and oxygen levels; and supports the removal of toxins from the organs that cause aging.

DRINK WATER TO RELAX

It is a known fact that water is great for everything from our internal organs to our skin.

But what has also been discovered is that it calms the nervous system, which holds the keys to balancing stress levels by conducting the traffic of electrical messages throughout the body.

When you are feeling a little scattered, the nervous system contracts and jumbled signals are given.

Drinking water immediately smooths out the jumbled signals through your whole body, which in turn calms the mind, so we can think more clearly.

Drink a glass of water slowly and feel yourself relaxing immediately.

Daily calming of the mind allows us to find a sense of stillness and in that we find a relaxed sense of happiness and a strong sense of our goodness as human beings.

It takes a lot of energy being something we are not, but it takes no energy to be yourself.

3

FOODS TO DELIVER HEALTHY SKIN, LOWER STRESS AND INCREASE TESTOSTERONE

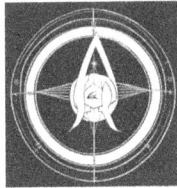

Body fat makes oestrogen, which can tip the ratio of oestrogen to testosterone to make testosterone levels unfavourably low.

D. ELIZABETH KAVALER, MD, UROLOGIST LENOX HILL HOSPITAL, NEW YORK CITY

STOP THE SKIN ATTACK

Food is one of the most powerful ways to help regenerate our skin, lower our stress levels and build our testosterone.

CORTISOL LOWERING FOODS

Healthy Fats help lower cortisol

You can't go wrong with a good fat. Omega-3 fatty acids are vital for skin health, but can also lower cortisol levels. Fish oil is known to lower cortisol levels and increase serotonin in the brain.

Other good fat sources include avocados, nuts and seeds, olive oil, egg yolks and...

- Goji berries
- Walnuts
- Sesame seeds
- Pumpkin Seeds
- Salmon
- Sardines
- Mackerel
- Anchovies
- Dark green lettuce
- Brazil nuts
- Extra virgin olive oil
- Sunflower oil
- Sesame oil

Magnesium reduces cortisol levels and is a muscle relaxant

Good sources of Magnesium include:

- Salmon
- Soybeans
- Brown rice
- Almonds
- Avocado
- Banana
- Green vegetables
- Spinach
- Milk
- Yoghurt
- Oatmeal

Vitamin C reduces the secretion of cortisol

Good sources of vitamin C include:

- Sweet red pepper
- Broccoli
- Strawberries
- Papaya
- Lemon (and other citrus fruits)
- Brussels sprouts
- Cantaloupe
- Tomato
- Cucumber

Protein in the diet can help reduce cortisol production

Protein-rich foods are often a good source of vitamins and minerals, which supports the overall health of skin.

These include fish, eggs, meat, poultry, dairy and foods such as soybeans, rice, pea, hemp and vegetable proteins. But the good news is that protein will not only reduce the stress hormone cortisol but will simultaneously power up the health of your skin and your T-levels.

Vitamin B Complex helps reduce cortisol

Vitamin B Complex has a variety of B vitamins that are great for the skin and is used by the body when it is under stress. Good sources of group B vitamins include:

- All lean meats
- Fish
- Chicken
- Turkey
- Eggs
- Organ meats (kidney, liver)
- Prawns
- Milk (and other dairy products)
- Almonds
- Seeds
- Beans
- Green leafy vegetables
- Carrots
- Turnips
- Celery
- Rice bran
- Soy

Low-glycemic carbohydrates can also support the body to lower cortisol levels naturally

Make sure to avoid sugary carbohydrates that can lead to insulin surges, which cause body fat storage.

Lower glycemic foods include:

- Vegetables
- Sweet potatoes
- Brown rice
- Whole wheat bread and pasta
- Beans

Cortisol surges after intense physical activity so be sure to eat a serve of carbohydrates immediately after you have done some exercise.

FOODS THAT BUILD TESTOSTERONE & HEALTHIER SKIN

You will see that most of the testosterone building super foods are on the list, so you will be able to create your own eating plan that not only builds testosterone, but lowers cortisol at the same time.

Any testosterone building diet should include foods that are high in vitamins D, B and minerals zinc and magnesium, incorporated into a cortisol lowering regime and eating plan.

To build testosterone naturally it will be important to include high levels of phytonutrient rich fruit and vegetables and minimise your sugar intake, which stimulates insulin and cortisol production.

Also avoid foods with soy as it can lead to an increase in oestrogen levels, which impacts testosterone levels.

Good fats and clean proteins are important, so ensure that you include olive oil and omega 3 fatty acids in your diet.

As testosterone levels fluctuate from morning to night, intermittent fasting is also known to support higher testosterone levels. So, try to leave at least 12 hours and up to 16 hours between your last meal and breakfast a few times a week.

These super foods are known to support the building of testosterone.

- Oily fish
- Shellfish
- Onion
- Garlic
- Ginger
- Spinach
- Green leafy vegetables
- Cruciferous vegetables
- Eggs
- Oysters
- Extra virgin olive oil
- Almond
- Honey
- Asparagus
- Avocado
- Pomegranate
- Banana
- Porridge oats
- Lemon

Foods high in Zinc include:

- Lean meat
- Dairy
- Shellfish
- Eggs
- Yogurt
- Nuts
- Seeds
- Legumes – chickpeas and lentils

Foods high in vitamin D include:

- Oily fish such as salmon, sardines and tuna
- Oysters and shrimp
- Eggs
- Mushrooms

THE BENEFITS OF THE MIGHTY CUCUMBER TO COUNTERACT THE IMPACTS OF STRESS

There are a number of superfoods that support our skin, but cucumber is worth calling out purely because of its versatility as one that supports the skin inside and out, while also supporting the body to lower stress and reduce toxins.

HANGOVER PREVENTION – Eat half a cucumber before going to sleep. Cucumbers reduce the nasty symptoms of hangovers because they contain a combination of B vitamins and enough natural sugar and electrolytes to help replenish many of the essential nutrients that are lost with high alcohol consumption.

ELIMINATE TOXINS - Cucumbers are ninety-five percent water, keeping the body hydrated while helping the body eliminate toxins.

NATURAL VITAMIN PILL - Cucumbers have many of the vitamins the body needs in a single day. Don't peel them because the skin contains a good amount of vitamin C - approximately 10 percent of the daily-recommended allowance, which is great for collagen production.

ENERGY BOOST - Cucumbers are a good source of B vitamins. So, if you need a quick energy boost, reach for a cucumber instead of that coffee in the afternoon

BYE BYE BAD BREATH - Take a slice of cucumber and chew it slowly, ensuring it reaches the roof of your mouth. The phytochemicals will kill the bacteria in your mouth responsible for causing bad breath.

AIDS IN DIGESTION - The high water content and dietary fibre in cucumbers are very effective in ridding the body of toxins from the digestive system, while aiding digestion.

I might not be exactly where I want to be but I am thankful that I have moved on from where I used to be.

4

FOODS TO AVOID

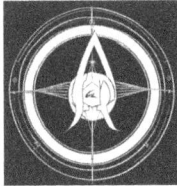

The best recommendation would be balance in your diet, limiting processed foods, particularly refined carbohydrates like sugar and get adequate sleep.

DR. ROBERT MORDKIN, CHIEF UROLOGIST
VIRGINIA HOSPITAL CENTRE

While many foods help regenerate our skin, lower our stress levels and build our testosterone, the opposite is also true. The food and beverages that we ingest can have a negative impact on our skin health and cause skin dryness.

This means they should only be consumed in moderation:

- Caffeine
- Alcohol
- Excess salt
- Overly spicy foods
- Soy
- Sugar

Worrying about tomorrow does nothing productive but destroys your sense of peace today.

5

THE IMPACT OF SUGAR ON THE SKIN

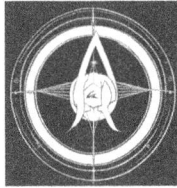

If you are serious about skin health and maintaining skin vitality over a lifetime, reduce your sugar intake.

GREGORY LANDSMAN

One of the staples of a Western diet is sugar, yet consuming sugar rich foods or beverages is one of the very worst things we can do for our skin.

Consuming sugar in any form increases blood sugar levels in the body, which promotes the 'glycation' process in our skin. Glycation damages our skin's collagen, causing it to become less elastic and more rigid, which in turn increases lines and wrinkles.

This means that anything we eat or drink that spikes our sugar levels is having a negative impact on the texture and quality of our skin.

So, while you might be in the habit of enjoying donuts, cakes, and energy drinks, these are major skin offenders - as are protein bars, flavoured yogurt, cereal and most sauces that come pre-made in a jar. These might look healthy, but are sugar tornados that create chaos with our skin.

Also keep in mind that low fat foods are often low in fat and high in sugar, which is bad for your skin on two levels:

1. High sugar levels cause glycation and reduce skin elasticity; and
2. The skin needs a moderate amount of 'good fats' in the diet to remain plump and elastic.

So, anything that is low in fat and high in sugar is drying and damaging every part of your skin from the inside out.

Dealing with life's challenges doesn't create character, it reveals it.

PART 2

SKIN HACKS FOR DRY SKIN

6

SKIN HACKS TO STOP THE SKIN ATTACK AND DE-STRESS

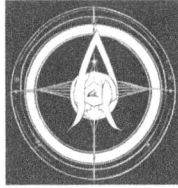

Stress is a full body physiological phenomenon, and your skin is an innocent bystander that gets swept up into the conflict. In addition to making you feel frantic and overwhelmed, the neurological and hormonal effects of stress wreak havoc on your skin. Stress induced adrenaline surges can cause wrinkles, acne and dullness.

DENNIS GROSS, M.D., DERMATOLOGICAL
SURGEON NEW YORK

SKIN HACKS TO ADDRESS DRY SKIN TOPICALLY

Our 'go to' solution for dry skin on any part of the body is usually applying some form of moisturising agent.

Moisturisers usually come in the form of creams and lotions, which are called emollients – substances that soften rough, dry or flaky skin; filling cracks in the skin caused by dryness and dehydration and soothing the skin.

The most commonly used emollients are lotions and creams.

LOTIONS

Lotions are predominantly made up of water with only a small amount of oil content. They are less moisturizing than creams but will always spread easily as they are generally quite thin in their consistency. Most lotions contain preservatives and chemicals and rarely feature any solid nutrients that contribute to the underlying health or strength of the skin's dermis.

CREAMS

Creams are made up of oil and water. This makes them easy to spread on your skin, but they don't have enough oil based ingredients to trap water in the skin. While a cream will always spread easily and feel good when you put it on, this doesn't mean that it is feeding your skin the nutrients it needs or contributing to building the strength of the skin – which is essential to combat skin dryness and make it more robust when exposed to lifestyle factors that dry the skin. It also means that it needs to be constantly reapplied, as the moisturising effect doesn't last.

The reality is that most creams and lotions feel good in the short term, but they are providing short term relief to the symptoms of dry skin, rather than providing a real solution.

OCCLUSIVES AND SLUGGING THE SKIN

I think by now we can safely conclude that there are many things in our environment working against men's skin. Because the uncomfortable symptoms of dry skin, (cracking, microtears, irritation, flaking etc.), are often the result of the moisture skin barrier being compromised and no longer able to hold the moisture required to maintain healthy skin, we need to stop the attack by sealing in moisture so it can start to repair.

Slugging skin is the practice of covering the skin in an occlusive skin product – one that is oil based and locks in the moisture and hydration in the skin. This improves the skin barrier and helps stop further damage to the skin.

We also need to provide the skin with the skin renewing vitamins and minerals that it needs to restore and repair. So ideally slugging is done with an occlusive formula that delivers high levels of skin nutrients in the form of skin building vitamins and minerals to support the skin to stay healthier and plumper.

Keep in mind that the most effective occlusives are 100% natural and enriched with vitamins that support and renew skin health. Slugging with creams or formulas that are full of artificial fragrances and preservatives and chemical toxins can increase underlying skin dryness and irritation.

WHY NATURAL SKIN HACKS WORK

While we have access to so many potions and lotions promising great results, the fact is that science shows that some of the most powerful skin boosting ingredients are 100% natural and can be found in your kitchen.

SOME OF THE MOST POWERFUL SKIN BOOSTERS FOUND IN YOUR KITCHEN AND USED FOR TOPICAL APPLICATION

Alpha Hydroxy Acid (AHA) acts as a natural exfoliant that removes dead skin cells and leaves skin healthier and renewed. AHA can be found in a number of foods and plants in different forms including glycolic acid, malic acid, lactic acid and citric acid.

Glycolic Acid is one of the most effective AHAs used for skin exfoliation, oil reduction, collagen building and skin bleaching. It can be found in sugar (from sugar cane) and unripened grapes.

Lactic Acid gently exfoliates and softens the skin and can be found in dairy products.

Malic Acid is also good for skin exfoliation and can be found in nectarines, bananas, cherries, blackberries, apples, pears and grapes.

Vitamin A (made up of Retinol and Carotene) renews skin through the stimulation of elastin and collagen production, resulting in smoother, more elastic skin. It has been shown to remove fine lines, repair sun damage and reduce age spots.

Vitamin A is found in egg yolk, milk and other dairy products, fish, fish oil, sweet potato, carrot, raw spinach, raw tomato, papaya, apricot, broccoli, orange and cantaloupe.

Vitamin C is known to stimulate collagen production, which gives the skin elasticity. It helps neutralise free radical activity, protects against UVA / UVB rays and helps heal scar tissue and bruising.

Vitamin C can be found in citrus fruits, peaches, strawberries, cranberries, mangos, green and red peppers, papaya, pineapple, grapes, mustard greens, broccoli, cabbage, spinach, tomatoes, fortified cereals, berries, melons, potatoes, kiwi, guava, peas, sweet potato and parsley.

Vitamin E is known to condition and moisturise the skin, inhibit free radical damage and help heal scars.

Vitamin E can be found in wheat germ, nuts, sunflower seeds, vegetable oil (including olive, safflower, sunflower), green leafy vegetables, tomatoes and whole grains.

Vitamin B3 helps regulate oil secretion and decreases a pre-disposition to blemishes. It can prevent dermatitis and scaly skin and is known as an acne treatment.

Vitamin B3 is found in cranberries, tomatoes and green peas. These foods can be used as a pulp to make a mask that can be applied to the face for 20 minutes.

Vitamin B5 helps to increase moisture content in hair and skin. Vitamin B5 is found in cranberries, sunflower seeds, tomatoes, strawberries, yoghurt, whole eggs and winter squash.

Vitamin D has strong moisturising properties and encourages tissue development. Vitamin D can be found in egg yolk, salmon, liver, herring, fortified milk and sunflower oil.

WHERE TO FIND SKIN BOOSTING INGREDIENTS

Aloe Vera
Aloe Vera is moisturising and soothing to the skin and regenerates healthy skin cells. It contains vitamins C, A, E and B and a series of minerals, enzymes and amino acids which are known to be anti-inflammatory.

Apple cider vinegar
Apple cider vinegar keeps skin supple. It's heavy concentration of enzymes helps peel off dead skin cells. Use as an astringent on oily skin.

Avocado
The oil in avocado tightens the skin and penetrates the layers to the deepest level. It is good for reducing fine lines and enhancing overall skin tone. Avocado contains more than 25 essential nutrients and vitamins, including high levels of vitamins E and C, which stimulate collagen production.

Baking Soda
Baking soda is a natural exfoliant, neutraliser and skin soother.

Banana
The antioxidants and nutrients in bananas help to restore collagen in your skin. They also have antibacterial properties and can be applied to the face mashed with lemon (stops the banana going brown), or with yoghurt, honey, egg or milk for a range of benefits that assist in maintaining skin health.

Barley
Barley is full of antioxidants and enzymes together with vitamins A, B, C and E. It helps elasticity in the skin and is both regenerative and moisturising.

Carrots
Carrots are an excellent source of vitamin A which is essential in the maintenance of healthy skin and hair, as well as Coenzyme Q10 (also found in many high quality face creams).

Citrus Fruit
Citrus fruits contain vitamin C (collagen building) which helps neutralise free radical activity and most importantly promote collagen synthesis – the key to skin remaining youthful and elastic.

Cucumber
Cucumber contains vitamins A and C (collagen building), and is a strong antioxidant with a number of trace minerals and enzymes essential for skin growth and repair. It is a good

source of silica, a trace mineral that contributes to the strength of connective tissue. Cucumber is immediately effective on puffy eyes, sunburn or as a tonic for the whole face.

Eggs
Eggs contain vitamins A, B5 and D, and proteins that have a tightening and constricting effect on the pores of the face. When egg whites are used as a mask they remove dead skin cells. Used as a hair rinse, the proteins in the eggs condition the hair follicles, leaving them smoother and shinier.

Epsom Salts
Epsom salts or Magnesium Sulphate is a long time remedy that has a multitude of benefits when applied topically or used for soaking. Epsom salts have a high magnesium content and is a natural muscle relaxant that can assist in lowering blood pressure, reducing stress, improving sleep and calming the nervous system. In a bath the salts draw toxins through the water and absorb the nutrients through the skin. Epsom salts are associated with helping back pain and aching limbs and also treating cold and congestion through the release of toxins.

Grapes
Grapes are high in AHA (skin renewal) and vitamin C (collagen building), so they are powerful for use as a skin exfoliant, for oil reduction on the skin and skin bleaching.

Honey
Honey both attracts and retains moisture and is soothing and nourishing to the skin. It contains a natural exfoliant and is

hydrating and calming to sore or irritated skin. Honey can be used for all over body nourishment in a range of treatments.

Lemon
Lemons are rich in AHA and vitamin C (collagen building) and a range of nutrients that has ensured its use as a rejuvenating beauty product for hundreds of years. Its versatility as a topical ingredient means it can be used in cleansers, toners, skin lighteners, face masks and scrubs. It is naturally antiseptic and has been used successfully to treat fine lines, scars and pigmentation of every kind.

Milk
Milk and yoghurt soften and soothe the skin because of the presence of lactic acid (AHA), a gentle exfoliant which renews and hydrates skin. High in vitamins A and D, milk nourishes and soothes dry, itchy and irritated skin, holding natural properties that calm irritation and reduce redness.

Oatmeal
Oatmeal is appropriate for dry and sensitive skin, acting as both an exfoliator and moisturiser.

Olive Oil
Olive oil is extremely high in vitamin E and vitamin K (found in green leafy vegetables), and contains high anti-oxidant and anti-inflammatory properties that help counteract exposure to pollution, smoke and alcohol. Olive oil is so rich in its nutrient value that it can be used topically on any part of the body to moisturise and regenerate.

Orange

Orange is high in vitamins A and C (collagen building), and of great benefit to all skin types via its regenerative skin properties. Orange stimulates circulation and the release of toxins from the skin.

Papaya

Papaya is high in AHA that removes the top layer of dead cells and helps regenerate fresh new skin. It also contains vitamins C (collagen building), E and K which support overall skin health.

Peach

Peach is a great source of antioxidants that help protect your skin from UV rays. Research has shown that nutrients from topically applied juice benefit the strength and elasticity of skin.

Pineapple

Pineapple is a citrus fruit (vitamin C – collagen building), which contains high levels of AHA, has a hydrating effect on the skin and is anti-inflammatory - the overall result is one that promotes clearer looking skin.

Potato

Potatoes contain vitamins C (collagen building), and B and minerals such as potassium, magnesium, phosphorus and zinc – all of which are good for the skin. Potato juice is excellent in skin packs and can assist in curing pimples and spots on the skin. It can also provide immediate relief from burns if placed directly on the area. Potatoes are also a skin cleanser and natural skin lightener.

Rose Water
Rose Water stimulates skin, balances pH levels, tightens pores and increases blood flow. It is antibacterial and appropriate for dry and oily skin.

Sugar
Sugar contains glycolic acid that is part of the AHA family, which helps break down dead skin cells leaving skin renewed and revitalised. Sugar can be applied topically to the face or the whole body as a scrub that hydrates skin without clogging pores.

Tea
When applied topically the tannins in tea reduce inflammation. Tea is known for putting oxygen into the skin and fighting free radicals that are destructive.

Tomatoes
Tomatoes are rich in vitamin A, vitamin C (collagen building), and potassium, essential for fresh glowing skin.

Turmeric
Turmeric is a natural antibiotic, a strong antioxidant and anti-inflammatory, and acknowledged as a potent anti-aging ingredient.

Vegetable Oils
Oils such as apricot kernel, avocado, almond, peach kernel, jojoba, sunflower, sesame, olive or soybean are all rich in unsaturated fatty acids, vitamins and minerals that are essential to maintenance of moisture levels in the skin.

Vinegar

Vinegar can help restore the natural pH balance in your skin, which assists with dryness, itching and flaking. It can be used as a cleanser and toner for your skin when mixed with water.

Watermelon

Watermelon is high in the super antioxidant lycopene and vitamins C (collagen building), A and B, which keep the skin fresh, radiant and hydrated. The natural acids act as an exfoliant, which are good for removing blemishes.

Yoghurt

Yoghurt contains AHA (skin renewal), vitamins A and B5 and will act as a gentle exfoliant that increases the moisture content in skin and hair. It will also cool and soothe irritated skin.

Balance is the act of life

Enthusiasm is the energy of life

Acceptance is the art of life

Understanding is the process of life

Trust is the faith in life

You are the essence and reflection of life

7

DE-STRESS YOUR FACE

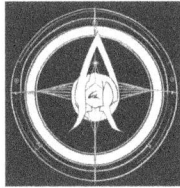

The skin and the central nervous system are intertwined, Therefore, it's not surprising that almost any and all skin diseases can be impacted by changes in the nervous system. Stress especially can leave a mark.

DR. ADAM FRIEDMAN, DIRECTOR OF
DERMATOLOGIC RESEARCH AT MONTEFIORE
MEDICAL CENTER NEW YORK.

EARLY MORNING MASSAGE

First thing in the morning give it a good hard rub, get the blood pumping, release and let it go!

Massaging your face speeds up lymphatic drainage, which removes toxins and de-stresses the muscles on the face and neck that cause lines, a sagging jawline, heavy jowls and frown lines.

This routine can be done first thing in the morning or last thing at night before the contraction movements.

Step 1: Before you start, rub hands together vigorously and place over the face to energise.

Step 2: Oil is required to provide a thin surface for hands to glide over, so the skin is not pulled or stretched.

Step 3: With all of the reviver movements, work upwards. This way the veins benefit most from the blood circulation created through this process.

Step 4: Start with a slow speed and increase the speed as you go, ensuring that the skin has only slight pressure placed on it. Be aware that as you do the massage, your skin may appear red or slightly blotchy immediately afterwards. This simply shows that it is working and that there is additional circulation in the area.

Step 5: Breathe deeply and slowly and you will feel your facial muscles relax. Let each breath empower you and let go of the stress and tension.

TOOLS TO BANISH FOREHEAD WORRY LINES

There is no doubt about it; our lifestyle and environmental stresses all take their toll on our skin.

But here are numerous natural treatments to hydrate, counteract, remove and prevent worry lines. Here are some home remedies to obtain a smoother, firmer, younger forehead.

1. Gently exfoliate your forehead once a week with 1 teaspoon of brown sugar, mixed with 1 tablespoon of olive oil. Rinse off with warm water
2. Rub a slice of potato over your forehead every morning and every night or alternate with some cucumber juice.
3. Apply your moisturiser and give your face and forehead a good massage. This speeds up the lymphatic drainage system and oxygenates the blood.
4. For a quick skin boost, rub an ice cube over your forehead furrows for less than a minute to improve blood circulation and help prevent forehead lines.
5. Use sun protection and avoid smoking.
6. Drink a minimum of 8-10 glasses of water a day to hydrate the skin and help flush the toxins that age the skin.
7. Massage the forehead, using three fingers to rub the forehead upwards from the brows to the hairline in a continuous movement.

When you feel comfortable in your skin you are able to feel comfortable in life, so regardless of what people or life throws at you, it doesn't stick.

8

REVITALISE THE FACE

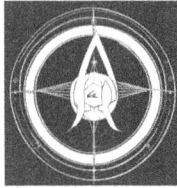

When the body is free of worry and stress, hormone levels remain relatively balanced. But when faced with conditions that are psychologically or physically stressful, the body's "flight or fight" response is triggered, and the sympathetic nervous system sends signals to the adrenal glands to flood the system with adrenaline and cortisol, both major stress hormones. As a result, the skin suffers from the body's chemical responses to psychological stressors. The skin – the human body's barrier against the damaging effects of the outside world – is less able to act as a shield.

DR. CARLA MARIE GRECO, CLINICAL
PSYCHOLOGIST, SANTA ROSA, CALIFORNIA

EXFOLIATION FOR MEN'S SKIN

If your skin is looking dull, lifeless and lack lustre then this treatment will kick start the circulation and improve the tone and condition of your skin by removing a build up of dead skin cells and pore clogging impurities. Keeping your skin exfoliated is one of the big keys to wake up your skin.

This weekly treatment is great if you are time poor. I always advise male models to use this treatment, especially when they are travelling on location or after a long day. It is one of the easiest ways to revive tired, stressed skin and is a powerful treatment that fits with every lifestyle.

METHOD:
Step 1: Splash cool water onto your face to wake up the circulation.
Step 2: Sprinkle a couple teaspoons of baking soda into the palm of your wet hand, adding drops of water as necessary to form a smooth paste.
Step 3: Gently smooth all over the face and massage the paste in small circular motions to exfoliate, but do not rub around the eye area.
Step 4: Rinse completely with cool to lukewarm water.
Step 5: Pat dry and follow with a moisturiser.

This is an exfoliant, so if your skin is highly sensitive dissolve a couple of teaspoons of baking soda in a cup of water and rinse your face with it rather than rubbing in circular motions.

THE SKIN SCIENCE:
Sodium bicarbonate smooths skin and is derived from a naturally occurring mineral that can help regulate and neutralize acidic or alkaline pH levels.

POTENT ULTRA SKIN RENEWING NIGHT SERUM AND DEEP PORE CLEANSER

If your skin is finding it hard to keep up with your hectic lifestyle, this treatment will wake up, defend and de-stress weary skin.

Step 1: Add 3 tablespoons of almond oil and ½ teaspoon of apple cider vinegar to an airtight dark glass bottle.

Step 2: Shake well before use.

This should make enough for one cleansing and moisturising treatment.

TO CLEANSE AND TONE:

Step 1: Apply the serum to the face.

Step 2: Take a warm face cloth and wipe over the skin.

TO MOISTURISE:

Step 1: Take the same serum and apply a few drops onto a damp face.

Step 2: Massage serum onto the face and neck in circular upward motions, giving your face and neck a firm massage as it tones, strengthens and nourishes the facial muscle fibres.

THE SKIN SCIENCE:
This concentrated blend feeds your skin vital nutrients.
Almond oil is full of oleic acid and vitamin E which is skin
regenerating, reducing the appearance of wrinkles and fine
lines. Apple cider vinegar contains polyphenolic antioxidants
that improve skin's appearance and citric acid, an alpha
hydroxy acid that exfoliates, smooths and brightens skin.

5 MINUTE SKIN BOOSTER MASK

This treatment is like boot camp for our skin and works hard
to keep the skin fit and healthy.

METHOD:
To make the powerful anti-oxidant skin treatment, all you
need is 2 tablespoons of Manuka honey.
Step 1: Apply the honey to the face and leave on for 15
minutes.
Step 2: Wash off with a warm cloth.
Step 3: Apply moisturiser to a damp face.

THE SKIN SCIENCE:
Manuka honey is rich in natural vitamins and minerals that
help create the capillaries and tissues that produce collagen
fibres under your skin. It is loaded with antibacterial,
antioxidant, and anti-inflammatory properties to help purify
skin, while hydrating it.

GIVE YOUR SKIN A LIFT WITH AVOCADO

This super fat delivers more than just skin food! It is loaded with monounsaturated fats, minerals and vitamins - particularly B6, that will not only give you skin a boost, but your energy as well!

The purity and goodness of the avocados creamy textured flesh delivers amazing results.   Avocados are rich in anti-oxidants, and loaded with fatty acids, which work together to plump up the skin and smooth out fine lines. So the next time you eat an avocado don't throw the skin away.

METHOD:
Step 1: Peel the avocado and take three slices.
Step 2: Use your fingers to apply it evenly over the face.
Step 3: Take the outside skin of the avocado and use it to gently rub the paste into your skin. This gently stimulates and exfoliates at the same time.
Step 4: Leave on for fifteen minutes and rinse off with warm water.

This wrinkle-fighting mask is simple to make, but delivers maximum impact. Your skin will feel more toned, re-texturized and energerised and you have a skin boosting cream that is natural, pure and good for your skin.

THE SKIN SCIENCE:
Avocados are rich in antioxidants, and loaded with fatty acids, which work together to plump up the skin and smooth out fine lines.

GREEN TEA EYE BAG TREATMENT

A simple, pure and powerful revitalising eye treatment to combat fatigue, free radicals and dark circles.

So perhaps you have had one too many late nights, unexpected deadlines, or exposure to environmental toxins that stress the skin around the eyes, leaving them puffy with dark circles.

So what's a man to do?

METHOD:
Step 1: Reach for green tea bags and steep two of them in a cup of hot water for 10 minutes.
Step 2: After you have drunk the tea, which is chock full with antioxidants with great anti-aging properties, take the cool tea bags and place them over your eyes for 10-15 minutes.

These bags are loaded with powerful tannins that help shrink swelling and reduce the fluids around the eyes.

THE SKIN SCIENCE:
The tannins in tea reduce inflammation. Tea is known for putting oxygen into the skin and fighting the destructive free radicals.

LIP SERVICE

Okay, so you have primed, polished and slicked your hair for that special date, but if your lips are feeling harder than nails and have more cracks than an old footpath, then you might end up with a kiss on the cheek!

The skin on your lips is sensitive and exposure to the elements can leave them looking and feeling dry, cracked and burning.

The reason for this is that your lips don't have oil glands, so they don't have a natural in-built moisturiser or the melanin to provide protection against harmful UV rays.

METHOD:
Step 1: To protect and resurrect your lips, take an old toothbrush and dip it in a bit of olive oil.
Step 2: Gently brush your lips to remove the dead skin and soothe the cracking.

Regular application of lip balm with a hint of SPF once a day will help keep your lips in great shape and ready for any occasion!

THE SKIN SCIENCE:
Olive oil is rich in nutrients that moisturise and regenerate.

Stay in your power, hold your values close and set boundaries. This is how you honour yourself and let people know what you stand for, and more importantly, what you won't stand for.

9

DETOX & DE-STRESS THE BODY

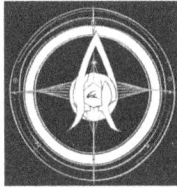

Psychological stress adversely affects the normal functions of the skin.

FLOR A. MAYORAL, MD, DERMATOLOGIST, FAAD,
UNIVERSITY OF MIAMI'S MILLER SCHOOL OF
MEDICINE

DETOX, DE-STRESS AND AGE LESS BODY TREATMENT

The food we eat is not the only factor that effects the aging process - stress and toxins can also cause premature aging.

Today we pack far more into our lives than ever before, demanding careers, hectic social lives, travelling and managing day-to-day challenges. The result is that many suffer from stress and an overload of toxins, which can age the skin and leave it dull, dry and lifeless.

So if you don't have the time to get to a health spa to detox and de-stress, you can get the same result with this ginger bath treatment. This skin detox bath stimulates circulation, opens the pores of the skin and eliminates toxins.

To make it you will need:

1 large nugget of fresh ginger
1 cup of Epsom salts
A muslin cloth and a ribbon or an old sock that is no longer in use.

Note: If you have sensitive skin or health concerns, consult your physician before trying this treatment. And do not take a hot bath if you have heart, or any other health issues.

METHOD:
Step 1: Grate the ginger into a bowl.
Step 2: Place the ginger in a muslin cloth or old stocking and tie it in a knot so that it becomes a ginger tea bag.
Step 3: While you are running the bath water place the

stocking in the bathtub and pour any juice from the bowl in as well.

Step 4: Add 1 cup of Epsom salts.

When you are ready to immerse yourself into the tub, leave the ginger infusion in the water while you soak. Allow at least forty minutes - the first twenty minutes helps your body remove the toxins, while the second 20 minutes are for absorbing the minerals from the water.

Ginger heats up the body and makes it sweat as you release toxins, so keep drinking water while in the bath so you stay hydrated.

Accumulated toxins age the organs and the body in general because they prevent our cells from regenerating efficiently. As well as ridding the body of toxins, a regular ginger bath helps regenerate the body and improve the complexion. It also helps the skin feel healthier and more toned.

For Super Dry Skin: After the bath, apply a light coating of olive oil to the skin.

THE SKIN SCIENCE:
Ginger contains powerful antioxidants that support the health of the skin. Soaking in magnesium rich Epsom salts helps boost magnesium levels, relax the muscles, and supports the body to regulate over 325 enzymes. It plays an important role in organizing energy production and the elimination of harmful toxins that can cause premature aging.

ALL CLEAR - COUNTERACT STRESS BREAK OUTS

Our skin does a lot to support us…it protects us, warms us and transmits the loving touch of the ones we love. But in the same way that you look after your car when it breaks down, it makes sense to show your skin some care when it breaks out! These treatments can work magic on blemishes.

VIAGRA RASH TREATMENT

To make it you need:

Apple cider vinegar
Virgin olive oil

METHOD:
Step 1: Once a day, wipe the impacted area with a diluted apple cidar vinegar and water solution (50/50).
Step 2: Immediately afterwards apply a light covering of olive oil over the area. Leave on.

THE SKIN SCIENCE:
Apple cider vinegar helps to cleanse the skin and peel off dead skin cells. Olive oil is high in vitamin E and vitamin K and contains high anti-oxidant and anti-inflammatory properties. Its rich nutrient value helps to moisturise and regenerate the skin when used topically.

BANANA FACE NOURISHER TO COUNTERACT BLEMISHES

To help control blemishes, use this every day until your skin has cleared.

METHOD:
Step 1: Take 1 banana skin and rub the inside of the skin over the face and neck and leave for half an hour.
Step 2: Rinse off with cold water.

THE SKIN SCIENCE:
This treatment nourishes your skin with antibacterial properties and sulphur to counteract blemishes and assist in restoring collagen.

HONEY SPOT TREATMENT

METHOD:
Step 1: Warm a little honey and apply to trouble spots.
Step 2: Wash off after 10 – 15 minutes.
Step 3: Apply regularly.

THE SKIN SCIENCE:
Honey has antiseptic properties and is high in vitamin C, D, E and B complex, which support skin healing.

SUNBURN RELIEF TREATMENTS

TEA BATH TREATMENT

METHOD:
Step 1: Brew up a large number of tea bags and leave to steep until strong.
Step 2: Mix tea in a shallow bath of warm water.
Step 3: Soak affected areas until the water cools.

THE SKIN SCIENCE:
The tea reduces inflammation, oxygenates the skin and fights free radicals.

ALOE VERA TREATMENT

METHOD:
Step 1: If you have access to an Aloe Vera plant, open a leaf to remove the gel and apply directly onto the sunburnt area.
Step 2: Alternatively, cucumber skin can also be used for skin irritations and sunburns, in the same way that Aloe Vera would be used because of its anti-inflammatory properties.

THE SKIN SCIENCE:
The Aloe Vera cools, soothes, moisturises and regenerates skin cells with healing vitamins A, C, E and B and minerals that are anti-inflammatory and antimicrobial.

RESTORATIVE HAND TREATMENTS

If your hands are feeling dry or rough, try these treatments to restore healthy, smoother feeling skin.

SUGAR AND OLIVE OIL HAND TREATMENT

METHOD:
Step 1: Take a teaspoon of sugar and a tablespoon of olive oil.
Step 2: Mix and pour over hands.
Step 3: Rub the front and back of hands together and in between fingers.
Step 4: Rinse with warm water.
Step 5: Pat dry and gently rub hands together.

THE SKIN SCIENCE:
Glycolic acid renews the skin surface and nurtures with vitamins E and K.

OLIVE OIL AND SALT HAND TREATMENT GLOVES

METHOD:
Step 1: Cover hands in olive oil and salt.
Step 2: Place hands in plastic 'surgical gloves' from the supermarket and leave on for 20 mins.
Step 3: Remove gloves and rinse hands in warm water.

THE SKIN SCIENCE:
Olive oil delivers an intensive treatment that will moisturise, regenerate and protect skin with vitamins E and K.

FOOT BATHS TO REGENERATE DRY SKIN

Regenerate and soften your feet by soaking them in a bathtub or plastic basin with warm water.

METHOD:
Step 1: To the warm water add a cup of Epsom salts and soak the feet for at least 10 – 15 minutes. The salt will help to smooth your feet, leaving them relaxed and revived.

Alternatively…
Step 1: Add 5 – 6 tablespoons of Epsom Salts to approximately 4 litres of water.
Step 2: Add half a cup of white vinegar.
Step 3: Mix all ingredients and soak feet in the solution. This relaxes and revives while also helping to prevent perspiration and foot odour.

THE SKIN SCIENCE:
Epsom salts restore the natural pH balance of the skin, while the high magnesium content is a natural muscle relaxant that draws out toxins and may assist in reducing stress, improving sleep and calming the nervous system.

The people in your life who genuinely want the best for you will always help you to walk your path, not place obstacles on it.

PART 3

PENILE SKIN HEALTH

10

IT'S TIME TO LISTEN TO WHAT YOUR PENILE SKIN IS TELLING YOU!

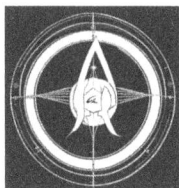

Your penis is a great barometer of overall health.

DR KEVIN BILLUPS, M.D. ASSOCIATE PROFESSOR
OF UROLOGY JOHNS HOPKINS MEDICINE

As men we listen to the news, we listen to our partners, we love listening to our favourite song, we even make time listen to our friends; but there comes a time in every man's life when he needs to listen to what his penis is telling him!

ONE OF THE BIGGEST IMPACTS ON PENILE SKIN HEALTH IS STRESS

Penile skin and it's functionality is a barometer for men's overall health and it won't hold back when it needs to tell you that you are suffering from stress overload.

Penile skin dries faster than any other area as it is thinner and more sensitive than most skin on the body. This makes it particularly vulnerable to the impacts of stress.

The upshot is - when you are stressed, so is your penile skin. The result is dry penile skin; micro tears; thinning skin; loose skin; and in many cases, cracked and peeling penile skin.

PENILE SKIN IS SUFFERING FROM DAY-TO-DAY LIVING!

We demand a lot from our penises but generally we take very little care of them. In many ways you might say that we take them for granted – expecting the penis to perform at peak fitness, without any real care.

Penile skin takes a beating everyday from normal daily activities and experiences. Some of these include:

Lubricants – Most men aren't in the habit of using skincare on the penis and so generally speaking the only application that is regularly applied to the penis area is lube. Most lubricants are full of skin drying chemicals. They are also largely water based and any water based commercially available skin product has preservatives in it to stop it growing bacteria. These preservatives also dry the skin. Constant exposure to skin drying chemicals takes a toll over time and makes penile skin dry, thinner and less elastic.

Soap – The genital area is generally doused in household soap at least once per day. Hot water and the chemicals in soap are harsh and remove the moisture barrier that keeps the skin on the penis healthy. This can lead to dryness, flaking and cracking and will make it more susceptible to skin infection due to the natural skin barrier having been weakened.

Lack of Air – The skin on the penis is rarely exposed to fresh air. Tight underwear creates friction on the skin and constricts the natural blood flow to the region. None of which is good news for penile skin health.

The Blue Tablet – It is important to be aware that several ingredients in the blue tablet are drying to the skin and in some cases can cause dryness, redness, scaling, or peeling of the skin (Mayo Clinic).

Dry damaged skin needs skin renewing vitamins and minerals to repair itself

When the moisture barrier of the skin is compromised by stress, low T-levels, lifestyle choices or just day to day living, the skin doesn't hold enough water and it dehydrates, leaving the skin vulnerable to cracking and flaking.

Medical peak bodies and academic institutions the world over acknowledge that toxins, lack of sleep and stress contribute meaningfully to premature aging of the skin and that prevention is supported by ingesting vitamins and minerals that feed the body and the skin.

Keep in mind that your skin absorbs whatever you put on it. The Dermatological industry has confirmed that using the right vitamins directly onto the skin can make a significant difference to maintaining healthier, younger looking skin; more so than merely taking vitamin tablets.

Vitamins are essentially antioxidants that work to neutralise damage from toxins within the deeper skin layers. And while vitamins work to counter the damage from toxins and skin stress, skin-building minerals are important for strengthening the connective tissue essential for stronger, fuller and more vital penile skin.

This is best achieved transdermally, through topical application directly on to the impacted skin in a way that maximises skin absorption and seals the skin barrier, stopping penile skin from drying and losing moisture.

Emollients vary enormously in terms of what they will contribute to the health of penile skin and their ability to deliver the vitamins and minerals it needs to combat dryness and pre-maturing aging of penile skin.

In men, the level of testosterone decreases with age. At the skin level, the result is observed as a decrease in density and lower elasticity.

PHILLIPPE BERNARD PHD BIOCHEMISTRY
UNIVERSITY OF ORLEANS, FRANCE

With low testosterone skin can become dry, and those with skin conditions such as psoriasis get worse.

UROLOGIST MIKE BUTCHER, DO, ANDROLOGY
FELLOW SOUTHERN ILLINOIS UNIVERSITY
SCHOOL OF MEDICINE

DRY AND IRRITATED PENILE SKIN TREATMENTS

INCREASE SKIN HEALTH WITH A FULL FAT YOGURT TREATMENT

Step 1: Generously apply natural full fat Greek yoghurt onto the penis.

Step 2: Leave on for ten minutes.

THE SKIN SCIENCE:
Yoghurt contains zinc, which is known for it's anti-inflammatory properties and facilitating tissue growth and cell production. It also helps with healthy skin renewal and preventing skin from dehydrating and drying. The B2, B5, B12 vitamins in yoghurt support healthy skin and the Riboflavin keeps the skin hydrated. The lactic acid in yogurt will help remove dead skin cells, while stimulating cells renewal.

REDUCE IRRITATION WITH A SOOTHING OATMEAL TREATMENT

Seal the deal with oatmeal and say goodbye to irritated, dry dull penile skin.

If you are looking for a quality ingredient that will deliver real results for dry, sensitive, irritated skin prone to dermatitis, psoriasis, and eczema, then you cannot go past oatmeal. This quick, effective treatment will calm irritated skin.

While you might recognise it as something good to eat for breakfast, the next time your penile skin feels like dried leather, it is time to make a skin deal with oatmeal!

You will need:

- 2 tablespoons rolled oats
- 1/2 tablespoon honey
- 2 tablespoons boiled water

METHOD:
Step 1: Put the oats into a blender and process into powder.
Step 2: Pour in hot water and honey. **Let it cool.**
Step 3: When cool massage the paste onto the penile skin.
Step 4: Leave on for 15 minutes.
Step 5: Remove with cool water.

THE SKIN SCIENCE:
Oats are loaded with Saponins, which are natural cleansers. It is full of healthy lubricating fats that prevent flaking and dryness and support the skin's natural barrier function, leaving it hydrated.

Honey is a natural humectant that holds water in the skin for maximum moisture and keeps skin looking moist and healthy.

Applying this treatment topically is an effective way to soothe irritated penile skin and eating it for breakfast is one of the easiest natural ways to increase testosterone in the bloodstream.

Life is too short to let your day-to-day happiness depend on how others respond to you.

11

SLUGGING PENILE SKIN

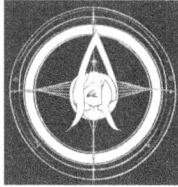

Moisturising adds back in to the skin the hydration needed to restore and maintain a healthier skin barrier. This makes the skin more resilient to the general aging processes.

DR DEAMBROSIS SPECIALIST DERMATOLOGIST

The symptoms of dry penile skin - cracking, microtears, irritation, flaking etc. - are often the result of the moisture skin barrier having been severely compromised and no longer able to hold the moisture required to maintain healthy penile skin. We can stop the attack by sealing in moisture, so it can start to repair.

THE BENEFITS OF SLUGGING

This can be done by slugging penile skin with an occlusive formula that delivers high levels of skin nutrients in the form of skin building vitamins and minerals to support the skin to stay healthier and plumper.

One of the best things you can do for your skin, is to slug skin and topically apply a natural oil-based, moisturising formula that is rich in vitamins and minerals to combat dry penile skin and contribute to penile skin health and vitality.

Regardless of whether you have oily skin or dry skin, it's important to moisturise your penile skin regularly. Using a 100% natural, fragrance-free moisturiser that's specifically designed to support penile skin can help prevent dryness; restore dry, irritated skin; and return the skin to its healthiest, fullest and most vital state.

It's never too late to be the best version of yourself.

12

PENILE SKIN HEALTH TIPS

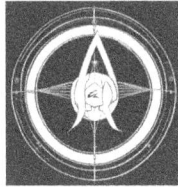

Small changes made regularly over time deliver BIG skin results.

GREGORY LANDSMAN

Dry penile skin is uncomfortable and something that most men experience at some point in their lives. We can minimise the drying and damaging impacts of our lifestyle choices in a number of ways, as the lifestyle behaviours that lower stress levels and maintain healthy testosterone levels, also naturally support healthy skin.

This includes the food we eat; our quality of sleep; mindfulness practices; and our day-to-day approach to exercise, water and counteracting the toxins we absorb in daily living.

Regardless of whether you are experiencing dry skin right now or are looking at strengthening and protecting your skin, it is important to practice regular penile self care.

LIFESTYLE TIPS THAT HELP COUNTERACT THE ATTACK AND CONTRIBUTE TO PENILE HEALTH

With that in mind here are some tips for counteracting the impacts of stress and lifestyle choices and keeping penile skin (and the skin on every part of your body) hydrated, vital and healthy:

1. **Avoid hot water**: Take warm showers and don't expose penile skin to hot water that compromises the skin moisture barrier.
2. **Avoid harsh soaps:** Soap can strip your skin of its natural oils. Look for mild, fragrance-free products that are formulated for sensitive skin.
3. **Choose your underwear carefully**: Avoid synthetic fabrics and wear loose underwear that allows your favourite organ to breathe.

4. **Cut down on sugar**: Minimise your sugar intake. Processed foods and food that is high in sugar can also contribute to inflammation and dryness in the body. Keep in mind that low fat products are often packaged up as healthy, but are in fact loaded with sugar.

5. **Focus on nutrition and maintain a healthy body weight**: Being overweight has an impact on blood flow, which is key to penile health. It also has an impact on testosterone levels, as when most men lose weight their T-levels naturally increase. Eat a balanced diet that is rich in nutrients and antioxidants. This helps support healthy skin, including the sensitive skin on the penis.

6. **Avoid food and drinks that dry the skin**: For example, spicy foods, caffeine and alcohol can all cause dehydration and irritation, which can exacerbate skin dryness and discomfort.

7. **Stay hydrated**: Drinking plenty of water throughout the day will keep you hydrated and help counteract skin dryness. Also try to eat food that has a high water content (such as fruits and vegetables), to keep you hydrated and promote healthy skin.

8. **Practice a daily relaxation technique**: Relaxation techniques such as deep breathing, meditation or yoga will help rid the body of day-to-day stresses.

9. **Exercise regularly**: Exercise moderately and regularly to boost your mood and reduce stress.

10. **Get enough sleep**: Prioritize sleep and aim for 7-8 hours of restful sleep each night.

11. **Practice good hygiene**: If the skin is cracked and has micro tears be sure to wash your hands before and

after touching your penis to prevent irritation and infection and avoid using harsh chemicals or fragrances in the genital area.

12. **Slug penile skin:** Use a vitamin rich occlusive moisturising formula to slug penile skin and strengthen skin health.

SMALL CHANGES CAN DELIVER BIG SKIN RESULTS

I suggest choosing a few things from the list above and then doing them regularly - as small changes over time can deliver big skin results. So if you do nothing else... these three changes will likely show your dry penile skin genuine improvement in a matter of days:

1. **Cut down on the harsh chemicals that your penile skin is exposed to;**
2. **Consume less sugar rich foods and drinks; and**
3. **SLUG penile skin daily with a good occlusive.**

Remember, your old self will remind you of the long distance you still need to go. Your new self will look at how far you have travelled to be where you are.

PART 4

SUPPORT FOR THE JOURNEY

13

SUPPORT FOR THE JOURNEY TO DE-STRESS & AGE LESS

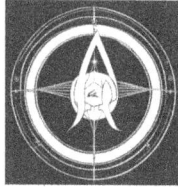

Lowering stress can help improve sexual function, decrease moodiness, and help men sleep better.

GREGORY LOWE, MD, UROLOGIST WEXNER
MEDICAL CENTER OHIO STATE UNIVERSITY

Here are a few suggestions that may support your journey to de-stress the body and the mind.

1. FISH OIL

Taking a good quality fish oil is important for overall skin health as the fatty acids will support testosterone production. Get odourless if you don't like the smell. Readily available online and at pharmacies and health food stores.

2. OMV One Manhood Vitamin – 100% natural topical skincare for slugging dry penile skin

For overall penile skin conditioning with vitamins and minerals, OMV is a scientifically proven occlusive formula developed to support dry penile skin and overall penile health. It features vitamins, minerals and fatty acids to support the natural building of testosterone. Perfect for slugging and endorsed by GQ. Available online and in selected pharmacies. See glskinfitinstitute.com

3. MASSAGE & REFLEXOLOGY

Regular massage and reflexology can support body relaxation and calmness.

4. BOOKS

CALM by Paul Wilson
Stop Stress Fast by Gregory Landsman
Don't Sweat the small Stuff…and it's all Small Stuff by Richard Carlson

5. MULTI B VITAMIN

Multi B vitamins support the nervous system during times of high stress.

6. VITAMIN D

Vitamin D is a key player in supporting and increasing the brain's serotonin levels - a chemical that helps reduce stress and anxiety and supports us to feel good. Ensure you are getting enough with a daily capsule; some very gentle early morning sun; or eating a diet rich in vitamin D with foods such as salmon, mackerel and tuna.

7. TEA

Chamomile Tea: Helps reduce stress and supports better sleep. Has great benefits in relaxing the muscles and reducing anxiousness.

Lemon Balm Tea: Calming and uplifting. It helps reduce the stress hormone cortisol and relax the body without causing drowsiness.

Green Tea: Contains an amino acid theanine, which helps promote relaxation and reduce stress.

Rose Tea: Helps reduce stress and supports good sleep.

8. ESSENTIAL OILS FOR STRESS & ANXIETY

The following essential oils may assist with lowering stress and calming the mind.

- **Lavender essential oil**: A tonic for the nervous system tonic that supports a balanced frame of mind.
- **Rose essential oil:** Can help relieve depression and anxiety.
- **Ylang Ylang essential oil**: Has uplifting and calming effects that support the nervous system.
- **Bergamot essential oil**: Helps in treating anxiety and depression.

- **Vetiver essential oil:** Is used in trauma and can support calmness.
- **Frankincense essential oil:** Supports feelings of calmness that help quiet the mind.

Something powerful emerges when we support each other to remember the truth of our humanity, the vulnerability of the human body and the strength of the human spirit.

14

GL DE-STRESS AND AGE LESS PRINCIPLES

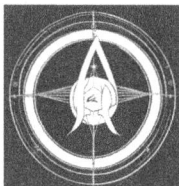

It is never too late to be all that you know you can be. So never discount your greatness.

GREGORY LANDSMAN

Practice wholeness - eat and exercise to increase the flow of energy and nurture wholesome emotions.

Breathe deeply, it supports your nervous system to relax and helps alleviate anxiety.

Put your heart into everything that you do and remain true to yourself.

Admire others, but never envy them.

Maintain a sense of humour and practice forgiveness.

Never argue for your limitations, only your possibilities.

Keep good company with yourself and practice sitting in silence for at least ten minutes every day.

Make peace with yourself by giving up self criticism and criticism of others.

Never judge others by their looks, as good looks do not necessarily equate to 'good people' or good love.

Learn to say 'no' to others and 'yes' to you. Never be scared to push back, as you train people how to treat you by what you allow them to do to you.

Give yourself permission to let emotions out of your body when feeling upset, rather than keeping them locked in. Allow yourself to feel it, so you can heal it.

Always choose to be kind and that also means approaching yourself with more kindness.

Let go of regret - we can't change our past but we can make peace with it and make different choices. When we know better, we can do better.

Concentrate on how you treat yourself, not on how others treat you. (Make sure you are not suffering from the 'disease to please others' at the expense of your own happiness!)

Always stand up for your individuality knowing that the key to your happiness is in holding deep convictions about who you are and what you believe.

Believe in your dreams and don't be afraid to follow them, even if no one else will. (Ask yourself regularly whether you are living the life you know you deserve, and if not, find ways to retrieve abandoned dreams and plans.

Remember your innate goodness as a person has nothing to do with your bone structure, but the structure of your thoughts and the way you choose to live and love on a daily basis.

Reminisce about things you loved to do as a kid and go and do some of them.

Recognise goodness in the things that you do, not only in the things you have.

Count your blessings and focus on what you have to give the world, rather than what the world has not given you.

Stay connected to nature (our greatest source of goodness), take a deep breath, kick off your shoes and feel the earth under your feet, feel the sun and smell the air.

Acknowledge every day that you are part of the miracle of life and at the end of each day spend a couple of minutes being grateful for that. The secret to having a positive outlook is seeing the good in the small things, such as the simple act of breathing, the smell of coffee or small acts of kindness from someone you love.

ABOUT THE AUTHOR

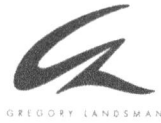

GREGORY LANDSMAN

Best selling author Gregory Landsman is one of the most noted beauty and wellness experts in the world and a best selling author of nine books on how to reduce stress (de-stress) and look younger (age less).

He is the host of the television program, Face Lifting Food, shown in more than 80 countries and the CEO of the GL Skinfit Institute; an organisation that creates innovative world class skin products to enhance skin health and defend it against environmental stressors and premature skin aging.

gregorylandsman.com

glskinfitinstitute.com

NOTES

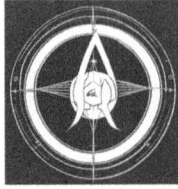

NOTES

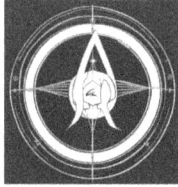

.

www.ingramcontent.com/pod-product-compliance
Lightning Source LLC
Chambersburg PA
CBHW051247020426
42333CB00025B/3093